Life-Saving Innovations: Advanced Techniques in Emergency Medical Services

Antoinette Kleinhans

Chapter 1: Introduction to Emergency Medical Services

The Evolution of Emergency Medical Services

The evolution of emergency medical services (EMS) has transformed significantly over the decades, reflecting advancements in medical knowledge, technology, and societal needs. Starting in the mid-20th century, the concept of pre-hospital care began to gain traction, initially characterized by basic first aid and transport methods. As communities recognized the importance of rapid medical intervention, the demand for more organized and efficient services grew. This period marked a pivotal moment, as it laid the groundwork for modern EMS, emphasizing the need for trained personnel who could provide care en route to medical facilities.

In the 1970s and 1980s, the establishment of national standards and protocols further shaped the EMS landscape. Training programs for paramedics and emergency medical technicians (EMTs) were developed, leading to a more skilled workforce capable of delivering advanced life support techniques. This era witnessed the introduction of advanced equipment, such as defibrillators and specialized airway management devices, which significantly enhanced the capability of EMS providers. The integration of these tools into everyday practice allowed for more effective interventions during critical situations, ultimately saving more lives and improving patient outcomes.

The design of ambulances has also undergone substantial innovation in response to evolving medical practices. Modern ambulances are now equipped with state-of-the-art technology, enabling them to serve as mobile emergency rooms. This includes advanced monitoring systems, communication tools, and storage for medications and supplies tailored for critical care. The shift from basic transport vehicles to fully equipped medical units reflects a broader understanding of the necessity for comprehensive care during transit, ensuring that patients receive continuous support while being moved to definitive care facilities.

Life-Saving Innovations: Advanced Techniques in Emergency Medical Services

Table Of Contents

Chapter 1: Introduction to Emergency Medical Services

The Evolution of Emergency Medical Services

The evolution of emergency medical services (EMS) has transformed significantly over the decades, reflecting advancements in medical knowledge, technology, and societal needs. Starting in the mid-20th century, the concept of pre-hospital care began to gain traction, initially characterized by basic first aid and transport methods. As communities recognized the importance of rapid medical intervention, the demand for more organized and efficient services grew. This period marked a pivotal moment, as it laid the groundwork for modern EMS, emphasizing the need for trained personnel who could provide care en route to medical facilities.

In the 1970s and 1980s, the establishment of national standards and protocols further shaped the EMS landscape. Training programs for paramedics and emergency medical technicians (EMTs) were developed, leading to a more skilled workforce capable of delivering advanced life support techniques. This era witnessed the introduction of advanced equipment, such as defibrillators and specialized airway management devices, which significantly enhanced the capability of EMS providers. The integration of these tools into everyday practice allowed for more effective interventions during critical situations, ultimately saving more lives and improving patient outcomes.

The design of ambulances has also undergone substantial innovation in response to evolving medical practices. Modern ambulances are now equipped with state-of-the-art technology, enabling them to serve as mobile emergency rooms. This includes advanced monitoring systems, communication tools, and storage for medications and supplies tailored for critical care. The shift from basic transport vehicles to fully equipped medical units reflects a broader understanding of the necessity for comprehensive care during transit, ensuring that patients receive continuous support while being moved to definitive care facilities.

Life-Saving Innovations: Advanced Techniques in Emergency Medical Services

Case studies of successful interventions during transit illustrate the impact of these advancements in EMS. There are numerous documented instances where timely and effective care provided by EMS teams has resulted in improved patient outcomes, particularly in cases of cardiac arrest or severe trauma. These interventions often highlight the importance of teamwork and communication among EMS professionals, which have become critical in achieving successful results. The ability to execute advanced life support techniques while en route has proven vital, showcasing the importance of ongoing training and adherence to best practices in emergency medicine.

Looking ahead, the future of emergency medical services will likely continue to evolve, driven by technological advancements and an ever-increasing understanding of patient care. Innovations such as telemedicine and artificial intelligence hold the potential to revolutionize how EMS operates, allowing for real-time consultations and enhanced decision-making in critical situations. As the field continues to adapt, the focus will remain on optimizing patient care and outcomes. The evolution of EMS is a testament to the dedication of professionals committed to saving lives and improving health care delivery in emergency situations.

Importance of Advanced Life Support Techniques

The importance of advanced life support techniques in emergency medical services (EMS) cannot be overstated. These techniques serve as a critical bridge between the onset of a medical emergency and definitive care at a hospital. Advanced life support (ALS) encompasses a range of sophisticated interventions, including advanced airway management, medication administration, and cardiac monitoring. By equipping emergency responders with these skills and tools, we significantly enhance patient outcomes during transit, reducing the likelihood of deterioration while en route to medical facilities.

Life-Saving Innovations: Advanced Techniques in Emergency Medical Services

Innovations in ambulance design play a vital role in the effectiveness of ALS. Modern ambulances are now equipped with advanced technology that supports critical care during transport. Features such as modular patient compartments, integrated monitoring systems, and advanced life support equipment ensure that paramedics can provide the highest level of care. These innovations not only improve the efficiency of emergency response but also enhance the safety and comfort of both patients and medical personnel. As design continues to evolve, we can expect even more effective solutions that cater to the specific needs of critically ill patients.

Case studies of successful interventions during transit illustrate the transformative impact of advanced life support techniques. For instance, in situations involving cardiac arrest, timely defibrillation and effective airway management can mean the difference between life and death. Documented cases highlight how quick, decisive actions taken by paramedics using ALS techniques have led to remarkable recoveries. These real-world examples serve not only as a testament to the efficacy of advanced life support but also as motivation for continuous training and improvement within EMS.

Moreover, the integration of technology into ALS practices is revolutionizing emergency medical response. Telemedicine, for example, allows paramedics to consult with emergency physicians while en route, facilitating real-time decision-making regarding patient care. This collaborative approach enriches the standard of care provided in transit, ensuring that patients receive expert guidance, which can be crucial in complex cases. As technology continues to advance, the potential for improved patient outcomes will only grow, underscoring the importance of ongoing innovation in ALS techniques.

In conclusion, the significance of advanced life support techniques in emergency medical services is clear. These techniques not only enhance the ability of responders to manage critical situations effectively but also reflect the ongoing commitment to improving patient care during transport. As we continue to explore innovations in ambulance design and integrate new technologies, the future of emergency medical services promises to be even more equipped to save lives, reinforcing the vital role of ALS in the continuum of care.

Overview of Innovations in EMS

The landscape of Emergency Medical Services (EMS) has undergone significant transformations in recent years, driven by a relentless pursuit of efficiency and effectiveness in life-saving techniques. Innovations in advanced life support techniques have emerged, enhancing the ability of paramedics and emergency responders to provide critical care in pre-hospital settings. These advancements not only improve patient outcomes but also empower EMS personnel with tools that allow for rapid assessment and intervention, ensuring that time-sensitive medical issues are addressed promptly.

One of the most impactful innovations in EMS is the integration of advanced monitoring technologies. Devices such as portable ultrasound machines and advanced cardiac monitors have become more prevalent, allowing for real-time diagnostics during transit. This capability enables paramedics to assess injuries and medical conditions with greater accuracy, ultimately guiding treatment decisions before patients reach the hospital. The ability to transmit vital signs and images to receiving facilities further enhances the continuum of care, ensuring that emergency departments are prepared for immediate action upon arrival.

In parallel, innovations in ambulance design have revolutionized the critical care environment on wheels. Modern ambulances are increasingly equipped with advanced life support systems, including integrated ventilation units and mobile infusion pumps. These enhancements ensure that patients receive continuous and comprehensive care during transport. Furthermore, the ergonomic design of the ambulance interior promotes better accessibility and workflow for EMS personnel, enabling them to perform complex procedures while minimizing the risk of injury or error.

Case studies of successful interventions in transit illustrate the effectiveness of these innovations. For instance, instances where paramedics utilized telemedicine to consult with specialists during transport have resulted in improved patient management for conditions such as stroke or trauma. These real-world applications highlight the importance of adopting cutting-edge technologies and strategies, demonstrating that timely decision-making and expert guidance can significantly alter patient outcomes in critical situations.

As EMS continues to evolve, the focus on integrating innovation into everyday practices remains paramount. Training programs are increasingly emphasizing the use of new technologies and techniques, ensuring that EMS personnel are equipped with the knowledge and skills necessary to adapt to these advancements. By fostering a culture of continuous improvement and embracing innovative solutions, EMS providers are better positioned to meet the dynamic challenges of emergency care, ultimately saving more lives and enhancing the quality of care delivered in the field.

Chapter 2: Advanced Life Support Techniques in Emergency Medical Services

Advanced Cardiac Life Support

Advanced Cardiac Life Support (ACLS) is a critical component of modern emergency medical services that significantly enhances patient outcomes during cardiac emergencies. This systematic approach provides a framework for healthcare professionals to respond effectively to cardiac arrest and other life-threatening cardiovascular conditions. By incorporating the latest clinical guidelines, ACLS emphasizes the importance of rapid assessment, high-quality cardiopulmonary resuscitation (CPR), and the timely use of advanced interventions. These innovations not only improve survival rates but also contribute to better neurological outcomes for patients who experience cardiac events.

One of the key features of ACLS is its reliance on a team-based approach, which facilitates the coordination of care among various providers. In an emergency, a well-organized team can quickly assess the patient's condition, initiate CPR, and determine the appropriate use of defibrillation and medications. The emphasis on teamwork ensures that all team members understand their roles and responsibilities, which is crucial in high-pressure situations. This collaborative effort is further supported by advances in training technologies, such as simulation-based learning, which enhances the preparedness of responders and fosters effective communication during critical interventions.

Recent innovations in ambulance design have further enhanced the delivery of ACLS in transit. Modern ambulances are equipped with advanced medical equipment, including portable defibrillators, advanced airway management devices, and comprehensive monitoring systems. These enhancements allow paramedics to perform advanced interventions en route to the hospital, thus minimizing the time to definitive care. The integration of telemedicine capabilities in ambulances also enables real-time consultation with emergency physicians, ensuring that treatment decisions are informed by the latest clinical data and guidelines.

Case studies of successful ACLS interventions in transit illustrate the profound impact of these advancements on patient outcomes. For instance, documented cases highlight instances where timely defibrillation and effective CPR during transport led to the survival of patients who otherwise would have faced dire consequences. These cases not only demonstrate the importance of ACLS education and training for emergency responders but also underscore the need for continuous improvement in prehospital care protocols. Learning from these successful interventions can inform future practices and drive innovations that enhance the efficacy of emergency medical services.

Life-Saving Innovations: Advanced Techniques in Emergency Medical Services

As the field of emergency medical services continues to evolve, the principles of Advanced Cardiac Life Support remain a cornerstone of patient care during cardiac emergencies. The integration of innovative technologies, enhanced training methodologies, and a team-centered approach ensures that responders are equipped to deliver life-saving interventions. By focusing on these advancements, emergency medical services can significantly improve patient survival rates and quality of life following cardiac incidents, ultimately fulfilling their mission to provide critical care in the most challenging situations.

Pediatric Advanced Life Support

Pediatric Advanced Life Support (PALS) is a crucial component of emergency medical services, particularly when it comes to the unique needs of children in critical situations. Unlike adults, pediatric patients have distinct physiological characteristics that require specialized approaches to assessment and intervention. The PALS curriculum emphasizes the importance of recognizing and managing respiratory and cardiovascular emergencies in children, ensuring that emergency responders are equipped with the knowledge and skills necessary to provide effective care in high-pressure scenarios.

One of the key innovations in PALS has been the development of age-appropriate resuscitation techniques and protocols. These protocols are informed by ongoing research and case studies that highlight successful interventions in pediatric emergencies. For instance, the integration of high-fidelity simulation training has allowed medical professionals to experience realistic scenarios that enhance their ability to respond swiftly and effectively. This hands-on approach not only builds confidence but also fosters teamwork among responders, which is vital in time-sensitive situations.

In addition to procedural advancements, innovations in ambulance design have significantly improved the delivery of PALS. Modern ambulances are now equipped with cutting-edge technology, such as advanced monitoring systems and pediatric-specific equipment, which facilitate rapid assessment and treatment during transit. These enhancements ensure that care providers can maintain close monitoring of vital signs and provide necessary interventions while en route to a medical facility, ultimately improving patient outcomes.

Moreover, case studies of successful PALS interventions during transport illustrate the effectiveness of these advancements. For example, a recent case highlighted a child experiencing severe respiratory distress who received immediate treatment with advanced airway management techniques while en route to the hospital. The integration of real-time communication between ambulance crews and hospital staff allowed for seamless transitions in care, demonstrating the importance of collaboration and preparedness in pediatric emergencies.

In conclusion, the evolution of Pediatric Advanced Life Support reflects a commitment to improving outcomes for young patients in critical situations. By embracing innovations in training, equipment, and collaborative practices, emergency medical services can enhance their ability to respond to pediatric emergencies effectively. As the field continues to evolve, it is essential for all stakeholders to remain informed and engaged in these life-saving advancements, ensuring that every child receives the best possible care when it matters most.

Trauma Management Techniques

Life-Saving Innovations: Advanced Techniques in Emergency Medical Services

Trauma management is a critical aspect of emergency medical services that requires a combination of established protocols and innovative techniques. In the high-stakes environment of trauma care, timely and effective interventions can mean the difference between life and death. Advanced life support techniques play a crucial role in stabilizing patients with traumatic injuries, and it is essential for emergency medical personnel to be well-versed in these methods. Techniques such as rapid sequence intubation, fluid resuscitation, and the use of tourniquets are fundamental to managing severe trauma. By mastering these skills, providers can optimize patient outcomes even before reaching the hospital.

Innovative ambulance designs are enhancing the capabilities of emergency medical services in trauma management. Modern ambulances are equipped with advanced medical technologies that allow for better monitoring and treatment during transport. Features such as integrated patient monitoring systems, automated CPR devices, and mobile imaging equipment can be life-saving tools in critical situations. These innovations not only improve the efficiency of care but also provide paramedics with the resources needed to perform advanced interventions in transit, bridging the gap between the scene of an accident and definitive care at a medical facility.

One of the key components of successful trauma management is the systematic approach to assessment and intervention. The use of the primary and secondary survey frameworks allows medical personnel to quickly identify life-threatening conditions and prioritize treatment. Training in these assessments is essential for all EMS providers, as it ensures that they can efficiently gather critical information and implement life-saving measures. Additionally, continuous education on the latest trauma management techniques and protocols is vital, as it empowers providers to stay current with evolving best practices and innovations in the field.

Life-Saving Innovations: Advanced Techniques in Emergency Medical Services

Case studies of successful interventions during transit highlight the importance of teamwork and communication in trauma management. Effective coordination among paramedics, emergency medical technicians, and dispatchers can significantly enhance the quality of care provided to patients. For instance, a case involving a multi-vehicle accident demonstrated how rapid communication facilitated the early identification of critical injuries and the allocation of appropriate resources. This collaborative approach not only improved patient outcomes but also showcased the effectiveness of innovative systems in place that support real-time decision-making during emergencies.

Looking toward the future, the integration of technology in trauma management will continue to evolve, fostering an environment where emergency services can respond more effectively to critical situations. Mobile applications that provide real-time data sharing, telemedicine capabilities, and advanced training simulations are just a few examples of how innovation can enhance trauma care. By embracing these advancements, emergency medical services can ensure that they are equipped to handle the complexities of trauma management, ultimately leading to improved survival rates and better overall patient experiences.

Innovations in Airway Management

Innovations in airway management have significantly transformed emergency medical services (EMS), enhancing both patient outcomes and the efficiency of care provided during critical situations. The advent of new technologies and techniques has provided emergency medical personnel with advanced tools to secure and maintain a patent airway, which is crucial in life-threatening scenarios. These innovations range from improved intubation devices to non-invasive ventilation methods, enabling responders to tailor their approach based on individual patient needs and circumstances.

Life-Saving Innovations: Advanced Techniques in Emergency Medical Services

One notable advancement is the development of video laryngoscopes, which offer enhanced visualization of the vocal cords compared to traditional laryngoscopes. This technology is particularly beneficial in difficult airway situations, where conventional methods may fail. With a video laryngoscope, paramedics can perform intubations with greater confidence and accuracy, leading to faster and more effective airway management. The integration of this technology into EMS protocols has reduced the incidence of complications associated with intubations and has been shown to improve overall success rates in the field.

Another innovation gaining traction is the use of supraglottic airway devices, which provide an alternative to endotracheal intubation, especially in scenarios where time is of the essence. These devices are easier to insert and can be utilized in pre-hospital settings with minimal training. Their design allows for rapid deployment, ensuring that oxygenation and ventilation can be maintained effectively while more definitive airway management is arranged. This flexibility can be particularly advantageous in dynamic environments such as ambulances and during transport to medical facilities.

Furthermore, advancements in airway management also extend to the development of portable ventilators and oxygen delivery systems designed for use in ambulances. These innovations facilitate high-quality respiratory support for patients experiencing respiratory distress, ensuring that they receive continuous care during transit. Enhanced monitoring capabilities integrated into these systems allow paramedics to observe vital signs and adjust ventilation settings in real-time, thereby improving patient outcomes during critical care transport.

Case studies of successful interventions highlight the impact of these innovations in airway management within EMS. Scenarios showcasing the use of video laryngoscopes and supraglottic airway devices demonstrate improved patient survival rates and reduced complications. As EMS continues to evolve, the adoption of these advanced techniques will likely play a pivotal role in shaping the future of emergency care, ensuring that patients receive the best possible interventions during their most critical moments.

Chapter 3: Innovations in Ambulance Design for Critical Care

Design Principles for Patient-Centric Care

Design principles for patient-centric care in emergency medical services (EMS) are essential to ensure that patients receive the highest quality of care during critical moments. The fundamental tenet of patient-centric design is to prioritize the needs and preferences of patients while delivering timely interventions. This approach requires a thorough understanding of the patient experience, which includes their physical, emotional, and psychological states during emergencies. By integrating these elements into the design of EMS protocols, equipment, and environments, care providers can foster a more supportive atmosphere that ultimately enhances patient outcomes.

One significant aspect of patient-centric design is the physical layout of ambulances and treatment areas. Innovations in ambulance design should focus on optimizing space for both patients and healthcare professionals. This includes creating modular spaces that can be easily reconfigured based on the patient's condition and the type of care required. Features such as adjustable lighting, noise reduction materials, and ergonomic equipment placement can help reduce anxiety and improve the comfort of patients during transport. Additionally, incorporating technology that allows for real-time monitoring and communication with hospital staff can streamline the care process and ensure that patients receive appropriate interventions as quickly as possible.

Another important principle is the integration of multidisciplinary teams in the decision-making process. By fostering collaboration among paramedics, emergency physicians, and specialists, EMS can ensure that care is tailored to the specific needs of each patient. This team-based approach allows for a comprehensive assessment of the patient's condition and facilitates a more informed strategy for care. Training programs that emphasize teamwork and communication skills are crucial in preparing EMS personnel to work effectively in high-pressure situations, ultimately contributing to better patient outcomes.

Cultural competence is also a key design principle in patient-centric care. EMS providers must consider the diverse backgrounds and needs of patients they encounter. This includes understanding cultural differences in responding to medical emergencies, as well as being sensitive to language barriers and varying levels of health literacy. Implementing training programs that focus on cultural awareness can equip EMS personnel with the tools necessary to provide respectful and effective care to all patients, ensuring that everyone feels valued and understood during their time of need.

Finally, feedback loops are essential for continuous improvement in patient-centric care. Establishing mechanisms for gathering patient and family feedback post-incident can provide invaluable insights into the effectiveness of care delivery and patient experiences. This data can then inform future design principles, training programs, and operational protocols. By fostering a culture of continuous learning and adaptation, EMS organizations can ensure that they remain responsive to the evolving needs of patients, ultimately leading to innovations that enhance the quality of care provided in critical situations.

Advanced Communication Systems

Advanced Communication Systems play a crucial role in enhancing the effectiveness of Emergency Medical Services (EMS), particularly in high-stakes situations where time is of the essence. The integration of sophisticated communication technologies allows EMS personnel to relay vital information quickly and accurately, ensuring that medical teams are prepared upon arrival at the scene or hospital. These systems facilitate real-time data sharing, enabling paramedics to provide critical updates about a patient's condition, treatment administered, and necessary resources required for optimal care. By streamlining communication channels, advanced systems not only improve response times but also enhance the overall coordination of care.

Life-Saving Innovations: Advanced Techniques in Emergency Medical Services

One of the most significant advancements in communication systems is the use of mobile data terminals (MDTs) and integrated dispatching software. These technologies allow EMS teams to receive instant updates and routing information, which is crucial in urban environments where traffic conditions can change rapidly. MDTs also enable paramedics to access patient records and data from previous calls, allowing for informed decision-making during emergencies. This access to information can be particularly beneficial in cases involving chronic illnesses or multiple medical conditions, where understanding a patient's history can significantly influence treatment decisions.

Furthermore, advancements in satellite communication and digital radio systems have vastly improved EMS communication capabilities, especially in remote or disaster-stricken areas where traditional networks may fail. These systems ensure that teams can maintain contact with dispatch centers and medical facilities, regardless of location or environmental challenges. The ability to communicate effectively in these scenarios is vital for coordinating multi-agency responses, facilitating a unified approach to patient care during disasters or mass casualty incidents. By leveraging these technologies, EMS providers can ensure that they are not only responsive but also resilient in the face of unpredictable circumstances.

Telemedicine has emerged as a pivotal component of advanced communication systems within EMS, allowing paramedics to consult with physicians in real-time. This capability significantly enhances the level of care provided during transit, enabling medical professionals to make informed decisions based on live assessments and expert opinions. The integration of video conferencing tools and mobile health applications into the EMS framework allows for immediate access to specialist advice, ensuring that patients receive appropriate interventions, even before reaching a hospital. This synergy between EMS and medical experts can lead to improved patient outcomes and can often be the difference between life and death in critical situations.

Lastly, the continuous evolution of communication systems in EMS is driven by the need for innovation and adaptability in an ever-changing landscape of healthcare challenges. The incorporation of artificial intelligence and machine learning algorithms into communication platforms is on the horizon, promising to enhance predictive analytics and optimize resource allocation. As these technologies develop, EMS providers will be better equipped to anticipate needs, improve operational efficiency, and ultimately save lives. By embracing these advancements, the EMS community can ensure that they remain at the forefront of emergency care, ready to respond to the complexities of modern medical emergencies with confidence and precision.

Modular Ambulance Concepts

The evolution of ambulance design has seen a significant shift towards modular concepts that enhance flexibility and efficiency in emergency medical services. Modular ambulance systems allow for the customization of various components based on the specific needs of patients and the types of emergencies encountered. This innovative approach not only optimizes the use of space and resources but also improves the overall quality of care provided during transport. By focusing on modularity, ambulance designs can better accommodate advanced life support equipment, ensuring that medical personnel have immediate access to essential tools and technologies.

One of the key advantages of modular ambulance concepts is their ability to adapt to different medical scenarios. For example, modular units can be configured to cater to trauma patients, cardiac emergencies, or pediatric care, allowing for quick modifications based on the situation at hand. This adaptability is crucial in critical care situations where time and efficiency are paramount. Moreover, the modular design facilitates rapid reconfiguration between calls, reducing downtime and ensuring that ambulances are always prepared for the next emergency, ultimately leading to improved patient outcomes.

In addition to flexibility, modular ambulance systems emphasize safety and ergonomics for both patients and medical staff. Advanced materials and design techniques are employed to create safe spaces that protect patients during transit, especially in high-impact situations. Furthermore, the layout of modular components is optimized for ease of access, enabling paramedics to work effectively in confined spaces while minimizing the risk of injury. This focus on safety and user-friendly design translates into better care delivery, as medical personnel can focus on their primary task—saving lives—without being hindered by the limitations of traditional ambulance designs.

Several case studies highlight the successful implementation of modular ambulance systems across various emergency medical services. For instance, cities that have adopted these concepts report higher satisfaction rates among paramedics and improved response times. In one notable case, a metropolitan area transformed its fleet with modular ambulances, resulting in a 20% increase in the number of patients treated on scene before transport. Such data underscores the tangible benefits of modular designs in real-world applications, paving the way for broader adoption in the field.

As the landscape of emergency medical services continues to evolve, modular ambulance concepts represent a promising frontier in improving critical care delivery. By embracing innovation and prioritizing adaptability, safety, and efficiency, the future of ambulance design can significantly enhance the effectiveness of emergency response teams. These advancements not only support the immediate needs of patients but also set a precedent for ongoing innovations in the realm of pre-hospital care, ultimately fostering a system that prioritizes life-saving interventions.

Integration of Telemedicine in Ambulances

Life-Saving Innovations: Advanced Techniques in Emergency Medical Services

The integration of telemedicine in ambulances represents a significant advancement in emergency medical services, enhancing patient care during transit. This technology allows paramedics and emergency medical technicians (EMTs) to connect with medical professionals in real-time, facilitating immediate access to expert guidance. By utilizing high-definition video feeds and secure communication channels, paramedics can relay vital signs, share images, and discuss treatment protocols with physicians and specialists, ensuring that patients receive informed care even before reaching a hospital.

Telemedicine systems in ambulances are designed to improve decision-making during critical situations. For instance, a paramedic encountering a patient with chest pain can transmit ECG readings to a cardiologist while en route to the hospital. This pre-hospital consultation allows for timely interventions, such as the administration of thrombolytics or the preparation of a catheterization lab upon arrival. By integrating telemedicine, ambulances become mobile treatment units, capable of initiating lifesaving procedures that can significantly improve patient outcomes.

The design of ambulances is evolving to accommodate telemedicine technologies, enhancing both functionality and patient comfort. Modern ambulances are equipped with advanced communication systems, including satellite connectivity and mobile data terminals, which ensure reliable connections even in remote areas. Additionally, user-friendly interfaces allow paramedics to operate telemedicine tools with minimal disruption to patient care. These innovations not only streamline operations but also create an environment conducive to effective medical interventions during transport.

Case studies of successful telemedicine interventions in transit highlight the technology's potential to save lives. In one notable instance, a rural ambulance team utilized telemedicine to stabilize a stroke patient by administering tPA treatment while en route to a medical facility. The ability to consult with a neurologist in real-time enabled the team to make critical decisions that significantly reduced the patient's risk of long-term disability. Such examples underscore the importance of integrating telemedicine into ambulance services, demonstrating how technology can bridge the gap between pre-hospital care and emergency department capabilities.

As the integration of telemedicine continues to evolve, the future of ambulance services looks promising. Ongoing advancements in technology, such as improved imaging tools and artificial intelligence algorithms, will further enhance the capabilities of paramedics in the field. By embracing these innovations, emergency medical services can not only improve patient outcomes but also set new standards for care delivery in the pre-hospital environment. This shift towards a more connected and informed approach to emergency care will undoubtedly redefine the landscape of ambulance services, making them indispensable in the quest for improved healthcare delivery in critical situations.

Chapter 4: Case Studies of Successful Interventions in Transit

Cardiac Arrest Interventions

Cardiac arrest is a critical emergency that requires immediate and effective intervention to improve patient outcomes. The cornerstone of cardiac arrest management includes early recognition, prompt initiation of cardiopulmonary resuscitation (CPR), and rapid defibrillation. Advanced Life Support (ALS) techniques, such as the use of advanced airway management and intravenous medication administration, play a pivotal role in enhancing the chances of survival. Innovations in training and simulation have empowered first responders with the skills necessary to perform these interventions effectively, ensuring that they can respond swiftly and confidently in high-pressure situations.

Life-Saving Innovations: Advanced Techniques in Emergency Medical Services

Innovative technologies have revolutionized the approach to cardiac arrest interventions. Automated external defibrillators (AEDs) have become commonplace in public spaces, allowing laypersons to deliver life-saving shocks before professional help arrives. Furthermore, advancements in wearable technology and mobile applications provide real-time data on a patient's condition, enabling emergency medical technicians (EMTs) to make informed decisions during transport. These tools not only facilitate immediate intervention but also streamline communication between first responders and hospital staff, enhancing the continuum of care.

In the realm of ambulance design, innovations have focused on creating a more efficient and effective environment for critical care during transport. Modern ambulances are equipped with advanced monitoring systems that track vital signs and provide data to medical personnel in real time. The layout of these vehicles has also been optimized to allow for rapid access to equipment and medications, reducing the time it takes to administer life-saving interventions. Such enhancements ensure that patients receive the highest level of care en route to the hospital, bridging the gap between pre-hospital and hospital care.

Case studies of successful interventions in transit underscore the importance of these advancements. One notable example involved a patient who suffered a cardiac arrest while attending a public event. The rapid deployment of an AED by bystanders, coupled with effective CPR and subsequent advanced interventions by paramedics en route to the hospital, resulted in a positive outcome. This case highlights the critical role of community preparedness, as well as the integration of innovative technologies and training, in saving lives during cardiac emergencies.

Life-Saving Innovations: Advanced Techniques in Emergency Medical Services

As the field of emergency medical services continues to evolve, ongoing education and training will remain essential. Incorporating the latest research and technological advancements into training protocols ensures that EMS personnel are equipped with the necessary skills to perform cardiac arrest interventions effectively. By fostering a culture of continuous improvement and embracing innovation, emergency medical services can enhance their response capabilities, ultimately leading to better survival rates and improved quality of care for patients experiencing cardiac arrest.

Stroke Response Successes

Stroke response successes highlight the critical advancements in emergency medical services that have transformed patient outcomes. The timely identification and treatment of strokes are pivotal in ensuring that patients receive the care they need as swiftly as possible. Innovations in communication technology allow first responders to relay vital information to hospitals, enabling pre-arrival notifications that prepare healthcare teams for immediate intervention. This proactive approach has not only reduced the time to treatment but has also significantly increased the chances of recovery for stroke patients.

Advanced life support techniques play a crucial role in the success of stroke interventions. Paramedics are now equipped with sophisticated tools and training that emphasize rapid assessment and intervention. The incorporation of portable imaging devices, such as ultrasound, allows for immediate evaluation of the patient's condition in the field. By identifying the type of stroke—ischemic or hemorrhagic—paramedics can initiate appropriate treatments, such as administering thrombolytics, before even reaching the hospital. This capability not only accelerates care but also enhances the overall efficiency of the healthcare system.

Life-Saving Innovations: Advanced Techniques in Emergency Medical Services

The design of modern ambulances has also contributed to the success of stroke responses. Innovations in ambulance design now prioritize critical care, offering advanced monitoring systems and specialized equipment that cater specifically to stroke patients. Features such as onboard telemedicine capabilities allow paramedics to consult with neurologists in real time, ensuring that critical decisions regarding patient care can be made during transit. This collaboration not only optimizes treatment plans but also empowers paramedics with the knowledge they need to make informed decisions.

Case studies of successful interventions in transit further illustrate the impact of these advancements. One notable example involved a patient experiencing severe stroke symptoms who was treated by a team that utilized both advanced imaging and telemedicine consultations. By confirming the diagnosis while en route to the hospital, the team was able to prepare for immediate surgical intervention upon arrival. This case exemplifies how the integration of technology and advanced techniques can lead to remarkable outcomes, highlighting the importance of continuous innovation in emergency medical services.

As the field of emergency medical services evolves, the successes achieved in stroke response serve as a beacon of hope and a model for other critical care scenarios. The commitment to improving patient outcomes through advanced life support and innovative ambulance design showcases the potential for further advancements in the field. By prioritizing timely and effective interventions, emergency medical services can continue to save lives and set new standards for excellence in healthcare delivery.

Trauma Victim Transport Innovations

Life-Saving Innovations: Advanced Techniques in Emergency Medical Services

Trauma victim transport innovations have revolutionized the way emergency medical services (EMS) respond to critical situations, ensuring that patients receive timely and effective care during transit. One of the most significant advancements in this field has been the integration of advanced life support techniques directly into ambulance design. Modern ambulances are now equipped with state-of-the-art medical technology that allows paramedics to perform life-saving interventions while en route to medical facilities. This seamless integration not only enhances patient outcomes but also empowers EMS personnel with the tools they need to stabilize patients during transport.

The design of ambulances has evolved considerably, with emphasis placed on creating an environment conducive to critical care. Innovations such as modular interiors allow for flexible configurations, accommodating various medical equipment and improving accessibility for healthcare providers. This adaptability ensures that emergency responders can quickly and efficiently use advanced life support equipment, such as ventilators and cardiac monitors, without compromising patient safety. Additionally, the incorporation of ergonomic features in ambulance design reduces the physical strain on paramedics, allowing them to focus on delivering high-quality care during high-pressure situations.

Communication technology has also seen tremendous advancements, facilitating real-time data sharing between EMS teams and receiving hospitals. Through the use of telemedicine and mobile applications, paramedics can transmit vital signs, imaging results, and other critical information while in transit. This proactive approach enables receiving facilities to prepare for incoming trauma patients more effectively, ensuring that appropriate resources are in place upon arrival. By streamlining communication, these innovations not only enhance patient care but also foster collaboration between EMS and hospital staff, ultimately improving overall trauma care systems.

Case studies of successful interventions during transport exemplify the impact of these innovations in trauma victim care. For instance, one notable case involved a multi-casualty incident where advanced pre-hospital care significantly improved survival rates. Paramedics utilized portable ultrasound devices to assess internal injuries in transit, allowing them to adjust treatment protocols and inform surgeons of specific conditions before the patients arrived at the hospital. Such interventions underscore the importance of equipping EMS with the necessary tools and training to respond effectively in critical situations.

As trauma victim transport continues to evolve, the focus remains on enhancing patient outcomes through innovative practices and technologies. Ongoing research and development in both ambulance design and advanced life support techniques are essential for addressing the dynamic challenges faced by EMS. By fostering a culture of innovation and collaboration, emergency medical services can ensure that trauma victims receive the highest standard of care, ultimately saving lives and improving recovery trajectories.

Maternal and Neonatal Emergency Cases

Maternal and neonatal emergencies represent critical situations that demand immediate and effective intervention. The complexity of these cases often stems from the unique physiological changes that occur during pregnancy and childbirth, as well as the vulnerabilities of newborns. Advanced Life Support Techniques (ALST) play a significant role in managing these emergencies, necessitating a thorough understanding of both maternal and neonatal needs. Innovations in ambulance design are also crucial, as they can enhance the efficacy of care provided during transit, ensuring the best possible outcomes for both mother and child.

In maternal emergencies, conditions such as hemorrhage, eclampsia, and obstructed labor require swift assessment and intervention. Emergency medical personnel must be equipped with the skills to perform rapid evaluations and initiate appropriate treatments. For instance, the administration of intravenous fluids and medications can be life-saving in cases of severe hemorrhage. Furthermore, the integration of point-of-care ultrasound technology in ambulances allows for quick assessments of fetal well-being and maternal health, enabling timely decision-making that can significantly impact outcomes.

Neonatal emergencies, including respiratory distress, congenital anomalies, and birth asphyxia, also require specialized attention. The use of advanced resuscitation techniques, such as positive pressure ventilation and chest compressions, can be critical in stabilizing a newborn. Training in these techniques is essential for emergency medical personnel, as the first few minutes of care are often decisive. Case studies illustrate how successful interventions, facilitated by well-prepared teams and appropriate technologies, can turn potential tragedies into positive outcomes, highlighting the importance of expertise and readiness in emergency situations.

Ambulance design plays a pivotal role in enhancing the delivery of care during maternal and neonatal emergencies. Modern ambulances are increasingly equipped with advanced medical equipment, tailored to the specific needs of pregnant women and newborns. Features such as adjustable stretcher systems, specialized lighting, and climate control ensure that both mother and child remain stable during transit. Furthermore, telemedicine capabilities enable real-time communication with specialists, allowing for informed decisions to be made while en route to healthcare facilities.

Ultimately, the intersection of advanced life support techniques, innovative ambulance design, and comprehensive training for emergency personnel creates a robust framework for managing maternal and neonatal emergency cases. As the field of emergency medical services continues to evolve, ongoing education and adaptation of new technologies will be essential. By embracing these innovations, we can ensure that both mothers and their newborns receive the highest standard of care during critical moments, paving the way for improved outcomes and survival rates.

Chapter 5: The Role of Technology in Emergency Medical Services

Wearable Medical Devices

Wearable medical devices represent a transformative advancement in emergency medical services, providing critical support in the assessment and management of patient care during transport. These innovative tools empower paramedics and emergency responders by enabling real-time monitoring of vital signs and other health metrics. By leveraging technology, these devices can transmit data directly to receiving hospitals, allowing medical teams to prepare for the patient's arrival and tailor treatment plans accordingly. This level of preparedness can be pivotal in high-stakes situations, where every second counts.

One of the primary benefits of wearable medical devices is their ability to continuously monitor patients' conditions. Devices such as smartwatches and specialized sensors can track heart rate, oxygen saturation, and even electrocardiogram readings. This continuous data flow provides paramedics with a comprehensive view of the patient's status, ensuring that any changes in condition are promptly addressed. Furthermore, the integration of these devices into ambulance design enhances the overall workflow, allowing for a more efficient response to emerging medical situations.

Life-Saving Innovations: Advanced Techniques in Emergency Medical Services

Innovations in ambulance design have also played a significant role in optimizing the use of wearable medical devices. Modern ambulances are increasingly equipped with advanced communication systems and docking stations for these devices, enabling seamless connections between the patient and healthcare providers. This integration allows for the efficient exchange of information, reducing the risk of data loss during transit. The design of ambulances now focuses not only on physical space for equipment but also on the technological infrastructure that supports these life-saving innovations.

Case studies of successful interventions using wearable medical devices illustrate their potential to improve patient outcomes significantly. For instance, instances where remote monitoring of cardiac patients during transport has led to timely interventions upon arrival at the hospital highlight the importance of constant vigilance. In these cases, the data collected contributed to quicker diagnoses and more effective treatment plans, demonstrating the vital role that wearable technology plays in emergency medicine. These real-world examples serve to inspire further integration of such devices into standard EMS practices.

The future of emergency medical services lies in the continued evolution of wearable medical devices and their integration into everyday practice. As technology advances, we can expect even more sophisticated devices that not only monitor but also provide feedback and predictive analytics to healthcare professionals. Training emergency responders to effectively utilize these tools will be crucial in maximizing their potential benefits. By embracing these innovations, emergency medical services can enhance patient care, improve outcomes, and ultimately save lives.

Drones in Emergency Response

Life-Saving Innovations: Advanced Techniques in Emergency Medical Services

Drones are revolutionizing the landscape of emergency response, offering unparalleled advantages in speed, efficiency, and accessibility. These unmanned aerial vehicles are now being deployed in various emergency situations, including natural disasters, medical emergencies, and search and rescue operations. The ability of drones to quickly survey large areas, deliver medical supplies, and provide real-time data is changing how emergency services operate. By integrating drone technology into emergency medical services (EMS), responders can enhance their capabilities and improve patient outcomes significantly.

One of the most compelling applications of drones in emergency response is their role in delivering essential medical supplies. In scenarios where traditional ground transportation faces obstacles due to traffic congestion or environmental hazards, drones can swiftly transport critical items such as defibrillators, blood products, or medications directly to the scene. This capability is particularly vital in rural or remote areas, where access to emergency care may be limited. By bridging the gap between patients and necessary medical interventions, drones ensure that time-sensitive treatments can be administered without delay.

Drones also play a crucial role in improving situational awareness during emergencies. Equipped with high-resolution cameras and thermal imaging technology, drones can provide real-time aerial views of disaster-stricken areas, enabling emergency responders to assess the scale of the situation quickly. This information is invaluable for coordinating rescue efforts, identifying hazards, and prioritizing resource allocation. Furthermore, drones can support search and rescue missions by scanning vast terrains and locating missing persons, ultimately saving lives when every second counts.

The integration of drone technology into ambulance design represents another innovative advancement in EMS. Some modern ambulances are now being equipped with drone deployment systems, allowing paramedics to send drones ahead of the vehicle to assess the scene or scout for safe landing zones. This proactive approach enhances the overall efficiency of emergency response, allowing crews to arrive on-site with a better understanding of the conditions they will face. As ambulance designs continue to evolve, incorporating drones as a standard feature will further streamline operations and improve the delivery of critical care.

Case studies from around the world highlight the successful implementation of drones in emergency response. In Sweden, for instance, drones have been utilized to deliver defibrillators to cardiac arrest patients, significantly reducing response times and improving survival rates. Similarly, in the United States, drones have been deployed to assist with disaster relief efforts, rapidly assessing damage and locating victims in the aftermath of hurricanes and wildfires. These examples showcase the transformative potential of drones in enhancing emergency medical services, paving the way for future innovations that prioritize patient care and save lives.

Mobile Applications for First Responders

Mobile applications have revolutionized the way first responders operate, providing them with real-time information and tools that enhance their ability to deliver critical care. These applications serve as both communication platforms and resource hubs, allowing emergency medical technicians (EMTs) and paramedics to access vital data quickly. Features such as GPS mapping, patient tracking, and medical protocol libraries enable first responders to make informed decisions on the scene, ultimately improving patient outcomes. The integration of mobile technology into emergency services represents a significant advancement in pre-hospital care.

Life-Saving Innovations: Advanced Techniques in Emergency Medical Services

One of the most impactful aspects of mobile applications for first responders is their ability to facilitate seamless communication among team members and other emergency services. This connectivity ensures that all personnel involved in a response are on the same page, which is essential during high-pressure situations. Applications can provide instant updates on the patient's condition, location, and treatment administered, allowing for a coordinated approach to care. By streamlining communication, these tools help mitigate the chaos that can often accompany emergency situations.

Additionally, mobile applications can serve as comprehensive medical resource libraries for first responders. They can include up-to-date treatment protocols, drug references, and guidelines for managing various medical emergencies. This access to information at their fingertips allows responders to adhere to best practices and make evidence-based decisions, even when faced with unfamiliar situations. The ability to consult a digital resource in real-time can be a game changer, especially in complex cases where time is of the essence.

Another significant benefit of mobile applications is their capacity for data collection and analysis. Many applications now include features that allow first responders to document patient assessments and interventions on the scene. This data can then be aggregated and analyzed to identify trends, improve protocols, and enhance training programs. By harnessing this information, emergency medical services can continuously evolve and adapt their practices based on real-world experiences, ultimately leading to improved care delivery in the field.

As the landscape of emergency medical services continues to evolve, the role of mobile applications is likely to expand further. Innovations in technology, such as artificial intelligence and machine learning, could enhance these applications, providing predictive analytics and personalized treatment recommendations. By embracing these advancements, first responders can be better equipped to handle the complexities of modern emergencies. The integration of mobile applications into the daily operations of emergency medical services not only enhances individual responder capabilities but also strengthens the overall effectiveness of the healthcare system during critical interventions.

Data Analytics for Improving Patient Outcomes

Data analytics plays a critical role in enhancing patient outcomes in the realm of Emergency Medical Services (EMS). By harnessing the power of data, healthcare professionals can make informed decisions that lead to improved care during emergencies. Advanced data analytics techniques allow for real-time assessment of patient conditions, enabling EMS teams to prioritize interventions effectively. This proactive approach not only enhances the quality of care provided in transit but also equips medical personnel with insights that can lead to better resource allocation and strategic planning.

One of the key applications of data analytics is in the identification of patterns and trends related to patient conditions. By analyzing historical data from various cases, EMS providers can develop predictive models that help anticipate patient needs based on specific indicators. For instance, tracking the frequency of cardiac events in certain demographics can inform targeted training for paramedics. This ensures that they are well-prepared to handle high-risk situations, ultimately leading to a higher likelihood of positive patient outcomes.

Moreover, advancements in ambulance design, influenced by data analytics, can significantly improve patient care during transit. By analyzing data related to patient movement, vital signs, and response times, designers can create more efficient ambulance layouts that enhance accessibility to critical equipment. These designs can incorporate features that facilitate better monitoring of patients, such as integrated technology for real-time vital sign tracking. As a result, medical teams can intervene more swiftly and effectively, ensuring that patients receive the necessary care as soon as possible.

Case studies of successful interventions highlight the transformative impact of data analytics on patient outcomes. Analyzing specific scenarios where data-driven decisions were made reveals that prompt identification of critical conditions often led to increased survival rates. For instance, a case study involving a multi-vehicle accident demonstrated how timely data analysis allowed EMS teams to prioritize the transport of the most critically injured patients to specialized trauma centers. These real-world examples serve as powerful testimonials to the importance of leveraging data for better decision-making in emergency situations.

In conclusion, the integration of data analytics into EMS practices is a vital component for improving patient outcomes. By utilizing data to inform training, enhance ambulance design, and guide clinical decisions in real-time, emergency medical personnel can deliver higher standards of care. As technology continues to evolve, so too will the methods by which data is collected and analyzed, paving the way for continuous improvements in emergency medical services. The commitment to embracing these innovations will ultimately lead to a more effective and responsive healthcare system capable of saving lives in critical moments.

Chapter 6: Training and Preparation for EMS Professionals

Simulation-Based Training Programs

Simulation-based training programs have emerged as a vital component in the education and preparedness of emergency medical services (EMS) personnel. These programs leverage realistic scenarios to provide hands-on experience in a controlled environment, enabling practitioners to develop critical skills without the high stakes associated with real-life emergencies. By immersing participants in lifelike situations, simulation training enhances their ability to respond effectively under pressure, ultimately improving patient outcomes during actual emergencies.

Life-Saving Innovations: Advanced Techniques in Emergency Medical Services

One of the primary advantages of simulation-based training is its ability to replicate complex clinical scenarios that EMS professionals may encounter in the field. These scenarios can range from advanced life support techniques to managing multiple casualties in a mass casualty event. By practicing these situations, EMS personnel can refine their decision-making skills, learn to prioritize tasks, and collaborate effectively with team members. This level of preparation ensures that when they face similar challenges in real life, they are equipped with the knowledge and experience to act decisively and efficiently.

In addition to clinical skills, simulation-based training programs also focus on innovations in ambulance design and critical care protocols. Participants can engage with the latest ambulance technologies, such as advanced monitoring systems and automated medication administration devices. This hands-on experience allows EMS professionals to familiarize themselves with new equipment and protocols, ensuring they can utilize these innovations effectively during transit. By integrating cutting-edge technology into training, programs prepare personnel not only to react but to leverage advancements that enhance patient care.

Case studies of successful interventions during transit further underscore the importance of simulation-based training. By analyzing real-life examples where EMS teams effectively employed their skills and knowledge, training programs can highlight best practices and areas for improvement. These case studies serve as valuable learning tools, allowing participants to explore what worked well and what could be enhanced in their own practice. This reflective learning process promotes a culture of continuous improvement within EMS teams, fostering an environment where innovation can thrive.

As simulation-based training continues to evolve, it holds the promise of transforming the landscape of emergency medical services. By embracing these programs, EMS organizations can cultivate a workforce that is not only technically proficient but also adaptable and resilient in the face of challenges. This commitment to ongoing education and innovation is crucial for advancing life-saving techniques and ensuring that emergency medical services meet the ever-changing demands of patient care in critical situations.

Continuous Education and Skill Enhancement

Continuous education and skill enhancement are vital components in the realm of emergency medical services, particularly within advanced life support techniques. As the landscape of emergency medicine evolves, practitioners must stay abreast of the latest protocols, technologies, and methodologies that can significantly impact patient outcomes. Regular training sessions, workshops, and certification programs not only keep EMS professionals informed about current best practices but also empower them to apply these innovations effectively in the field. The commitment to lifelong learning ensures that practitioners can respond with confidence and competence, even in the most challenging situations.

Innovations in ambulance design have created new opportunities for enhancing patient care during transit. Continuous education plays a crucial role in equipping EMS personnel with the knowledge to leverage these advancements fully. For example, understanding the functionalities of state-of-the-art equipment, such as advanced defibrillators and portable ultrasound machines, requires ongoing training. Familiarity with the latest designs, including improved ergonomic features and advanced communication systems, allows EMS professionals to optimize their response to emergencies, ensuring that they can deliver high-quality care while en route to medical facilities.

Case studies of successful interventions in transit highlight the importance of continuous education and skill enhancement. These real-world examples demonstrate how well-trained EMS teams have effectively utilized innovative strategies and technologies to improve patient outcomes. By analyzing these cases, practitioners can identify successful techniques and incorporate them into their training. This process not only fosters a culture of learning within the EMS community but also encourages the sharing of knowledge and experiences among peers, which is essential for professional growth.

Moreover, continuous education facilitates interdisciplinary collaboration, which is increasingly important in today's complex healthcare environment. By participating in joint training exercises with other healthcare providers, EMS professionals can better understand the roles and responsibilities of their colleagues in hospitals and other care settings. This collaboration ensures a seamless transition of care for patients, ultimately enhancing the quality of service provided. As EMS personnel enhance their skills and knowledge, they contribute to a more integrated healthcare system that prioritizes patient safety and effective communication.

In conclusion, continuous education and skill enhancement are indispensable for advancing emergency medical services. By embracing lifelong learning, EMS professionals can adapt to new challenges, utilize innovative technologies effectively, and collaborate with other healthcare providers to ensure optimal patient care. The commitment to ongoing training not only prepares individuals for the complexities of their roles but also fosters a culture of excellence within the EMS community, ultimately saving more lives and improving outcomes for those in critical need.

Team Dynamics in Critical Situations

In critical situations, effective team dynamics are essential for ensuring optimal patient outcomes in emergency medical services (EMS). The unpredictable nature of emergencies demands that team members not only possess advanced life support skills but also function cohesively under pressure. A well-coordinated response can significantly enhance the efficiency of medical interventions, leading to better survival rates and improved patient experiences. By fostering an environment of trust, communication, and mutual respect, EMS teams can navigate the complexities of critical care more effectively.

One of the key elements of successful team dynamics is clear communication. In high-stress scenarios, the ability to convey information succinctly and accurately can make a crucial difference. Team members must be trained to use standardized terminology and protocols to reduce misunderstandings. Regular training sessions that simulate realistic emergency situations can help teams practice their communication skills, enabling them to adapt seamlessly during actual interventions. Moreover, the use of technology, such as mobile communication devices and real-time data sharing, can further enhance coordination among team members, ensuring everyone is on the same page.

Collaboration is another cornerstone of effective team dynamics in EMS. Each member brings unique expertise to the table, and leveraging these diverse skills can lead to innovative solutions in critical care. For instance, paramedics trained in advanced life support techniques can work closely with emergency medical technicians who excel in logistical support, creating a well-rounded approach to patient care. Encouraging team members to contribute their insights during debriefings after interventions can foster an atmosphere of continuous learning and improvement, ultimately leading to higher standards of care.

Additionally, the physical environment of the ambulance plays a significant role in team dynamics. Innovations in ambulance design that prioritize teamwork can facilitate more efficient workflows. For example, ambulances equipped with modular layouts or adjustable workspaces can allow for better movement and collaboration during interventions. Such designs can also enhance the safety and comfort of both patients and crew, reducing stress levels and promoting a more effective response. Investing in ergonomic equipment and tools that are easily accessible can significantly improve the overall performance of the EMS team.

Lastly, cultivating resilience within the team is vital for maintaining optimal performance in critical situations. High-pressure environments can lead to burnout and fatigue, which can adversely affect decision-making and response times. Implementing wellness programs and mental health resources can help team members cope with the emotional toll of their work. Regular team-building exercises and support systems can strengthen relationships and foster a sense of camaraderie, ensuring that each member feels valued and supported. By prioritizing both individual well-being and collective strength, EMS teams can enhance their dynamics, ultimately leading to more effective interventions and better patient outcomes.

Stress Management Techniques for EMS Personnel

Stress management is crucial for EMS personnel, as they frequently face high-pressure situations that can lead to burnout and decreased performance. Implementing effective stress management techniques can enhance the well-being of emergency medical responders, allowing them to perform optimally during critical interventions. One of the most effective techniques is mindfulness meditation. This practice encourages individuals to focus on the present moment, reducing anxiety and improving concentration. By incorporating short mindfulness sessions into their daily routine, EMS personnel can cultivate resilience and maintain emotional balance, even in the face of challenging circumstances.

Physical fitness is another vital component of stress management for EMS personnel. Engaging in regular physical activity not only promotes overall health but also serves as a powerful stress reliever. Exercise releases endorphins, which can elevate mood and reduce feelings of stress. EMS agencies can support their staff by providing access to fitness programs or encouraging group workouts. Additionally, incorporating activities such as yoga or tai chi can offer EMS personnel tools for relaxation and self-regulation, enhancing both their physical and mental well-being.

Peer support systems play a significant role in managing stress within the EMS community. Establishing a culture of open communication among colleagues fosters an environment where personnel feel comfortable discussing their experiences and emotions. Regular debriefing sessions after challenging calls can provide a platform for EMS personnel to share their feelings and gain perspective from their peers. Creating structured support networks, including mentorship programs, can further enhance resilience by connecting less experienced responders with seasoned personnel who can offer guidance and encouragement.

Time management is a critical skill that EMS personnel must develop to combat stress effectively. The unpredictable nature of emergency medical services often leads to chaotic schedules and overwhelming workloads. By prioritizing tasks and setting realistic goals, EMS personnel can create a more manageable workflow. Utilizing tools such as digital calendars and task management apps can help responders keep track of their responsibilities and deadlines, reducing the feeling of being overwhelmed. Furthermore, learning to delegate tasks when appropriate can alleviate some of the pressure, allowing personnel to focus on their most critical duties.

Finally, promoting a healthy work-life balance is essential for long-term stress management in EMS personnel. Encouraging responders to take time off for self-care, family, and personal interests can prevent burnout and sustain high levels of motivation and performance. Agencies can implement policies that support flexible scheduling and provide resources for mental health support. By recognizing the importance of downtime and the need for personal rejuvenation, EMS organizations can create a healthier work environment that prioritizes the well-being of their personnel, ultimately leading to improved patient outcomes and enhanced service delivery.

Chapter 7: Future Trends in Emergency Medical Services

Advancements in Artificial Intelligence

Life-Saving Innovations: Advanced Techniques in Emergency Medical Services

Advancements in artificial intelligence (AI) have significantly transformed emergency medical services (EMS), enhancing the effectiveness and efficiency of healthcare delivery during critical moments. One of the most notable developments is the integration of AI algorithms in decision-making systems that assist paramedics in assessing patients' conditions in real time. These systems analyze vast amounts of data, including vital signs and medical history, to provide evidence-based recommendations. This capability not only improves the accuracy of diagnoses but also ensures that the most appropriate interventions are initiated promptly, ultimately saving lives.

In addition to diagnostic support, AI has revolutionized the logistics of ambulance design and operation. Smart ambulances equipped with AI systems can optimize routes based on real-time traffic data and historical patterns, ensuring that paramedics reach their destinations as quickly as possible. These vehicles can also monitor their own status and alert maintenance teams when repairs are needed, reducing downtime and improving overall readiness. As a result, the use of AI in ambulance design not only enhances critical care during transit but also maximizes the operational efficiency of EMS agencies.

AI's role extends beyond the confines of the ambulance, positively impacting patient outcomes through predictive analytics. By analyzing data from previous emergency calls and patient responses, AI systems can identify trends and forecast potential complications, allowing paramedics to prepare for specific cases before they arrive at the hospital. For instance, if a pattern emerges indicating a spike in cardiac events in a particular area, EMS can allocate resources accordingly and train personnel to focus on those scenarios. This proactive approach enhances preparedness and can lead to more effective interventions.

Moreover, case studies of successful interventions in transit highlight the tangible benefits of AI integration. In instances where real-time data from AI systems guided paramedics in administering life-saving treatments, outcomes improved dramatically. For example, AI-driven ECG analysis has enabled quicker identification of arrhythmias, facilitating timely defibrillation. Such innovations demonstrate that AI is not merely a theoretical concept but a practical tool that can be seamlessly woven into the fabric of emergency medical care, enhancing the capabilities of first responders and improving patient survival rates.

As the landscape of emergency medical services continues to evolve, the advancements in artificial intelligence are likely to play an increasingly pivotal role. The ongoing development and refinement of AI technologies promise to bring forth even more sophisticated tools that can aid EMS professionals in their mission to save lives. With a commitment to harnessing these innovations, the future of emergency medical services appears bright, characterized by enhanced decision-making, improved patient care, and a greater capacity to respond to emergencies effectively. This synergy of technology and human expertise will ultimately redefine the standards of care in critical situations.

The Impact of Virtual Reality on Training

The integration of virtual reality (VR) technology into training for emergency medical services (EMS) represents a transformative approach to prepare personnel for real-world scenarios. Traditional training methods often rely on simulations or static classroom environments, which can limit the realism of critical care situations. However, VR immerses trainees in lifelike environments where they can practice advanced life support techniques, hone their decision-making skills, and experience the pressures of a high-stakes emergency without the risks associated with real-life training. This immersive experience enhances retention and understanding, allowing EMS professionals to better translate their skills into actual practice.

Life-Saving Innovations: Advanced Techniques in Emergency Medical Services

One of the most significant advantages of VR training is its ability to replicate a wide range of emergency scenarios that EMS personnel may encounter in the field. From cardiac arrest to trauma cases, VR can simulate various environments, such as crowded public places or confined spaces, giving trainees the opportunity to develop their situational awareness and adaptability. This versatility ensures that EMS professionals are not only trained for the most common emergencies but are also prepared for less frequent but equally critical situations. By experiencing these scenarios multiple times in a controlled setting, trainees can build confidence and competence, which is crucial when every second counts in patient care.

In addition to enhancing technical skills, VR training fosters teamwork and communication among EMS crews. Effective collaboration is vital in emergency situations, and VR can create scenarios that require team members to work together seamlessly. By practicing in a virtual environment, EMS personnel can learn to verbalize their actions, share critical information, and coordinate their efforts under pressure. This training approach helps to break down barriers between team members, reinforcing the importance of clear communication and collaboration in delivering high-quality patient care during transport.

Moreover, the adaptability of VR technology allows for training programs to be tailored to the specific needs of various EMS organizations. Different regions may face unique challenges, such as varying patient demographics or geographical considerations. By customizing VR scenarios to reflect these specific contexts, EMS agencies can ensure that their personnel are adequately prepared for the types of emergencies they are likely to encounter. This targeted training approach enhances the overall effectiveness of EMS teams, ultimately leading to improved patient outcomes in critical care situations.

As VR technology continues to evolve, its potential applications in EMS training are expanding. Innovations such as haptic feedback and real-time performance analytics can further enhance the learning experience, providing trainees with immediate feedback on their actions and decision-making processes. As more EMS agencies adopt these advanced training techniques, the overall standard of care in emergency medical services will likely improve. By embracing virtual reality as a foundational element of training, EMS professionals can be better equipped to save lives and respond effectively in the face of emergencies.

Community-Based Emergency Response Models

In recent years, community-based emergency response models have emerged as vital components of effective emergency medical services (EMS). These models emphasize collaboration between emergency services, local organizations, and the community, fostering a more responsive and efficient system. By incorporating local resources and knowledge, these models enhance the overall capability of emergency response, ensuring that care is not only timely but also tailored to the specific needs of the community. This approach also encourages a sense of shared responsibility among citizens, empowering them to participate in their own safety and health outcomes.

One of the critical aspects of community-based emergency response is the integration of advanced life support techniques. Training local volunteers in basic life support and first aid can significantly improve survival rates in emergencies. These volunteers can act as immediate responders while professional EMS personnel are en route, bridging the critical gap that often exists in emergency situations. This model not only enhances the speed of care delivery but also alleviates some of the pressure on professional responders, allowing them to focus on critical cases that require advanced interventions.

Innovations in ambulance design have also played a significant role in the effectiveness of community-based emergency response models. Modern ambulances are increasingly equipped with advanced technology that facilitates rapid communication, real-time patient monitoring, and efficient space utilization for critical care interventions. These innovations ensure that EMS providers can deliver high-quality care even while in transit, maximizing the potential for positive patient outcomes. Community involvement in the design and operation of these ambulances can further enhance their effectiveness by ensuring they meet local needs and challenges.

Case studies of successful interventions in transit highlight the impact of community-based models. For instance, in several urban areas, partnerships between local health departments and community organizations have led to the development of rapid response teams that operate alongside traditional EMS units. These teams have demonstrated success in managing cardiac emergencies and trauma cases, often achieving better outcomes than traditional response models. By fostering collaboration and resource sharing, these innovative approaches have not only saved lives but also strengthened community resilience.

Ultimately, community-based emergency response models represent a paradigm shift in how emergency medical services operate. By leveraging local resources, enhancing training, and embracing innovative technology, these models create a more robust and effective emergency response system. As communities continue to face diverse challenges, the adoption and expansion of these models will be crucial in ensuring that emergency services remain responsive, efficient, and ultimately life-saving. The integration of community members into the EMS framework not only promotes a culture of preparedness but also reinforces the idea that public health and safety is a collective responsibility.

Shifts in Policy and Funding for EMS

Life-Saving Innovations: Advanced Techniques in Emergency Medical Services

Shifts in policy and funding for Emergency Medical Services (EMS) have become increasingly critical as the landscape of healthcare evolves. The growing demand for advanced life support techniques has prompted policymakers to reconsider the allocation of resources and the regulatory frameworks guiding EMS operations. These changes are vital for ensuring that EMS agencies can effectively respond to emergencies while integrating innovative technologies and methodologies. Increased awareness of the importance of timely and efficient emergency care has led to a push for enhanced funding mechanisms, enabling EMS providers to deliver higher-quality services.

Recent trends indicate a shift toward value-based funding models that emphasize patient outcomes rather than mere service volume. This transformation is encouraging EMS agencies to implement advanced life support techniques more effectively. By focusing on the quality of care delivered during transport, agencies can demonstrate their impact on patient survival rates and recovery, which can, in turn, attract more funding. Furthermore, this model encourages collaboration among EMS providers, hospitals, and community stakeholders to ensure that resources are allocated efficiently, promoting comprehensive care that extends beyond the initial emergency response.

Innovations in ambulance design for critical care are also being influenced by these policy shifts. As funding becomes more accessible, EMS agencies are able to invest in state-of-the-art vehicles equipped with the latest technology. These ambulances are designed not only to transport patients but also to provide advanced medical care en route. Features such as integrated monitoring systems, enhanced communication tools, and specialized medical equipment allow for better management of critical cases during transit. As policies evolve to support these innovations, the potential for improved patient outcomes increases, ultimately benefiting the healthcare system as a whole.

In addition to vehicle upgrades, changes in funding and policy have led to the development of comprehensive training programs for EMS personnel. As the demand for advanced life support techniques grows, so does the need for skilled professionals who can implement these practices effectively. New funding initiatives often prioritize education and training, enabling EMS providers to stay current with the latest advancements in medical care. This investment in human capital not only enhances the capabilities of individual EMS agencies but also contributes to a more knowledgeable and versatile workforce within the broader healthcare community.

The impact of these shifts in policy and funding is evident through various case studies of successful interventions in transit. These examples highlight how well-funded and well-equipped EMS teams can significantly improve patient outcomes, even in critical situations. By analyzing these successful cases, it becomes clear that a strategic approach to policy and funding can lead to transformative changes in emergency medical services. As stakeholders continue to advocate for better resources and innovative practices, the future of EMS looks promising, with the potential to save even more lives through sustained investments in advanced techniques and technologies.

Chapter 8: Conclusion and Call to Action

Recap of Key Innovations

In the rapidly evolving field of emergency medical services, key innovations have emerged that significantly enhance patient care and optimize responses during critical situations. One of the most notable advancements is the integration of advanced life support techniques, which have transformed how paramedics manage life-threatening conditions. Techniques such as high-performance CPR, the use of automated external defibrillators, and advanced airway management have become standard practices. These methods not only improve patient outcomes but also empower EMS personnel with the skills necessary to handle complex medical emergencies effectively.

Ambulance design has also seen remarkable innovations tailored to critical care needs. Modern ambulances are now equipped with advanced monitoring systems, state-of-the-art medical equipment, and ergonomic designs that facilitate easier access to patients. These vehicles include features such as adjustable lighting, climate control, and modular storage for medical supplies, allowing for a more organized and efficient response. Innovations like these ensure that emergency responders can provide high-quality care while minimizing the time spent on scene, thus enhancing the overall effectiveness of emergency medical interventions.

Furthermore, case studies of successful interventions in transit highlight the real-world impact of these innovations. For instance, the implementation of telemedicine in ambulances has allowed paramedics to consult with hospital physicians in real time, enabling immediate guidance on treatment protocols. This collaborative approach has proven invaluable in stabilizing patients before they reach the hospital, particularly in cases of trauma or cardiac arrest. Documenting these successful cases not only serves as an inspiration for EMS professionals but also reinforces the importance of continuous learning and adaptation in emergency medicine.

The role of technology in improving communication and data sharing cannot be overstated. Innovations such as electronic patient care reporting systems streamline documentation processes, allowing for better data collection and analysis. This advancement aids in the identification of trends and areas for improvement within EMS operations. Moreover, the use of mobile applications has empowered first responders to access vital information swiftly, enhancing decision-making in the field. This seamless integration of technology into emergency services has created a more informed and prepared workforce.

In conclusion, the recap of key innovations in emergency medical services demonstrates a commitment to enhancing patient care and operational efficiency. As advanced life support techniques continue to evolve, the design of ambulances adapts to meet the critical demands of the field, and successful case studies provide valuable insights for future practices. The ongoing integration of technology further supports improvements in communication and data management. Together, these innovations represent a significant leap forward in the capabilities of EMS, ultimately leading to better outcomes and saving more lives in emergency situations.

Encouraging Community Involvement

Encouraging community involvement in emergency medical services is vital for enhancing the overall effectiveness of care provided during critical situations. When communities actively participate in the development and implementation of emergency response strategies, they not only bolster the resources available to emergency personnel but also foster a culture of preparedness and resilience. By engaging local residents in training sessions, awareness campaigns, and volunteer opportunities, EMS organizations can create a network of informed citizens ready to assist in emergencies. This collaborative approach ensures that communities are not just passive recipients of care but active participants in their safety and well-being.

One innovative way to promote community involvement is through the establishment of Community Emergency Response Teams (CERTs). These teams can be trained in basic first aid, CPR, and emergency response techniques, empowering individuals to act effectively in crises. By providing structured training programs, EMS organizations can equip community members with the necessary skills to support professional responders during emergencies. Such initiatives not only enhance individual confidence but also create a sense of unity within the community, as members work together to prepare for potential disasters.

In addition to training, leveraging technology can significantly enhance community engagement. Mobile applications that provide real-time information on local emergencies, resources, and volunteer opportunities can keep residents informed and involved. For example, an app could notify users about local training sessions, upcoming emergency drills, and ways to volunteer in their neighborhoods. By making information accessible and fostering communication, EMS organizations can encourage a proactive approach to community safety, leading to a more prepared populace that understands the importance of their role in emergency situations.

Case studies of successful interventions highlight the positive impact of community involvement in emergency medical services. For instance, some communities have reported significant improvements in response times and patient outcomes when local volunteers were integrated into their EMS operations. These volunteers often provide crucial support, such as managing crowds, directing traffic, or assisting with basic care, which allows professional responders to focus on critical tasks. These examples serve as powerful reminders of the potential benefits that can arise from fostering collaboration between EMS providers and the communities they serve.

Ultimately, encouraging community involvement in emergency medical services is not just about enhancing immediate response capabilities; it is about building a culture of preparedness that extends beyond individual incidents. By fostering an environment where residents feel empowered to participate, EMS organizations can cultivate lasting partnerships that strengthen resilience and promote safety throughout the community. The commitment to encouraging such involvement reflects a progressive approach to emergency care, ensuring that every member of the community plays a vital role in safeguarding their collective health and well-being.

Vision for the Future of EMS

Life-Saving Innovations: Advanced Techniques in Emergency Medical Services

The future of Emergency Medical Services (EMS) is poised for a transformative evolution, driven by innovation and the relentless pursuit of improved patient outcomes. As technology advances and our understanding of emergency care deepens, the vision for the future of EMS encompasses enhanced clinical practices, streamlined operational efficiencies, and a deeper integration of technology. This vision is not only about adopting new tools but also about fostering a culture of continuous improvement and adaptation to meet the ever-changing demands of emergency care.

One of the key elements in this vision is the advancement of Advanced Life Support (ALS) techniques. The integration of cutting-edge medical devices and protocols can significantly enhance patient care during critical moments. Innovations such as portable ultrasound machines, advanced monitoring systems, and telemedicine capabilities will allow EMS providers to make more informed decisions while en route to medical facilities. This not only optimizes treatment but also ensures that patients receive the most appropriate care as soon as they arrive at the hospital, ultimately improving survival rates and recovery times.

In conjunction with advances in clinical techniques, the design of ambulances is also evolving to better meet the needs of critical care patients. Future ambulance designs will prioritize ergonomics, space optimization, and access to advanced technology. Vehicles will be equipped with modular systems that can adapt to the specific needs of different patients, allowing for a more personalized approach to emergency care. This innovation extends to the environment within the ambulance, where features such as improved lighting, noise reduction, and climate control will create a more conducive atmosphere for patient care and comfort during transit.

Case studies of successful interventions in transit will serve as invaluable learning tools for the EMS community. By analyzing instances where innovative techniques and technologies have been employed effectively, EMS providers can identify best practices and refine their approaches to emergency care. These case studies will highlight the importance of training and preparedness, showcasing how organizations that embrace a culture of learning and adaptation can achieve remarkable outcomes even in the most challenging circumstances.

Ultimately, the vision for the future of EMS is one where collaboration, innovation, and education come together to create a more efficient and effective emergency care system. By prioritizing advanced life support techniques, reimagining ambulance design, and learning from successful interventions, EMS will continue to evolve. This proactive approach will not only enhance the capabilities of emergency responders but also ensure that patients receive the highest standard of care during critical moments, fulfilling the promise of life-saving innovations in emergency medical services.

www.ingramcontent.com/pod-product-compliance
Lightning Source LLC
Chambersburg PA
CBHW051922250726
48659CB00002B/788